My P

Heartfelt Letters of Remarkable Healing with a Holistic Doctor

Dr. Danny Quaranto

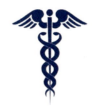

Medical Doctor (MD)
Doctor of Oriental Medicine (DOM)
Naturopathic Medical Doctor (NMD)

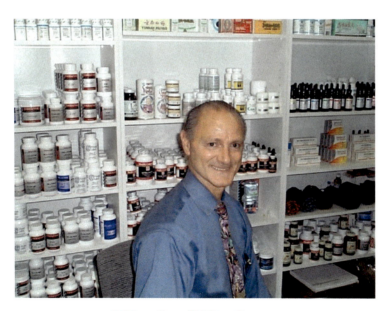

A Man for all Five Seasons

Copyright © 2016
lr032717

ISBN-13: 978-1533268853
ISBN-10: 1533268851

Pictures are in the public domain, used by permission, or labeled for reuse.

You can contact Dr. Danny at:

Alternative Medicine Family Care Center
2050 40th Avenue, Suite 2
Vero Beach, FL 32960
772-778-8877
DrDanny@amfcc.info
www.amfcc.info

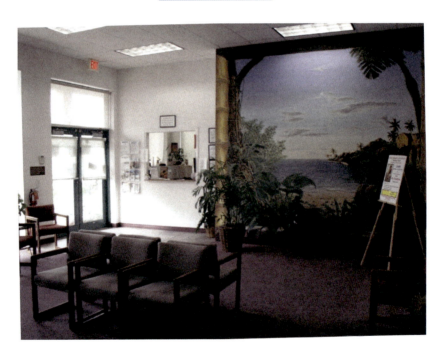

Contents

Foreword iv
Preface vi
Oriental Medicine 1
LETTERS FROM THE HEART 13
   Working with children 14
   Acupuncture 18
   Allergies 23
   Alternative medicine 26
   Arthritis 28
   Cancer 30
   Homeopathy 31
   Prolotherapy 35
   Pain Relief 37
   Smoking 41
   Surgery 42
   Vision, Eyes 43
   Other Ailments 44
MAKING LIFE WORTHWHILE 51
A MAN FOR ALL FIVE SEASONS 56
CONCLUSION OF THE MATTER 69
   A Patient Sums it Up 70
TAKING CONTROL OF YOUR HEALTH 71
ABOUT THE AUTHOR 77
   Acknowledgements 82
   Public Teaching and Health Videos 86

Foreword

By Kate Hoffmann

Acupuncture Physician
Doctor of Oriental Medicine
Former director of the Florida State
Oriental Medical Association

Acupuncture and Oriental Medicine has been around for about 3500 years. It has been used by half the world's population for everything that can and does go wrong with the health of people and animals. That means there is a plethora of techniques and modalities that have been found, tried, and 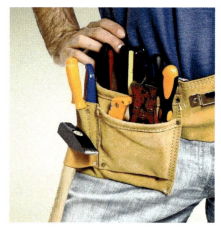 proven. And there are those health practitioners who include a large number of these tools in their tool belt in order to optimize the healing of their patients. Dr. Danny Quaranto is one of them.

Some people get better with age. While others make lists of what they want to do in retirement, Dr. Quaranto went back to school. Not just any school mind you, but medical school! He spent months with specialists during the rotations he undertook. He did more than needed in the dissection lab to more perfectly understand how the body works and uncover the secrets of this magnificent thing that we call our body. His Medical Doctor (MD) degree confirms his heartfelt and determined effort.

But why all this exertion? Simple. That he might restore more people to health and do so more effectively. That's a dedicated healer. As an example, when Christmas falls on Thursday, he is upset. Why? Because there are fewer days to help others.

If I want to know something about a technique, Dr. Danny has been to the class; he has read the book; he can tell me what it's about, and if it has helped his patients. He is the most passionate Acupuncture Physician/MD I have ever met. And as you will see in this book, his patients appreciate it. He has helped so many people in this town. He has put Acupuncture and NET (Neuro-Emotional Technique) on the map in Vero Beach.

Through his passion, kindness, and support, two young women, after working in his office in administrative positions, became acupuncture physicians. Now they are helping others. And he mentors many of his colleagues, including me.

He is kind and caring, carefully listening to his patients, which is integral to the art of healing. All this dedication that he might relieve suffering and restore health whatever the ailment may be.

Dr. Danny is a dedicated husband and father. He adores his wife and daughters. But his deepest passion is his clinic and his patients, restoring them as quickly as possible to optimal health.

I am honored to call him my mentor and friend. May he enjoy his work for many more years that his patients might continue to benefit from his extensive knowledge—and his kindness!

Preface

Why this book? Three reasons:
- That those already my patients might discover other areas in their lives in which they might receive help.
- That those not yet my patients might become inspired by hearing from those who have gone before.
- That those out of our area might use us as a resource to find a holistic practitioner local to them.

We are continually encouraged by patient stories (like family members really because that's how we feel after we come to know one another). They share with us the difference our care has made to their well-being. This begins with the health of the body, but to those who are willing, extends inward to the mind and emotions—even to the spirit.

We also appreciate the pat on the back about being kind and taking time to carefully listen. Everyone likes to know what they're doing has value and is appreciated. We thank you, our patients, for sharing your stories.

What follows are actual cases in which specific ailments were treated and lives changed. There's nothing like real-world experience to encourage you; what others have achieved, you can too.*

---

* The stories are as they were written, other than minor editing for readability and clarity.

You'll undoubtedly find your ailments portrayed and begin thinking how you too can heal and see a real difference in your life. If you don't find what concerns you, we no doubt have encountered it, so ask us.

The stories are as they were written, other than minor editing for readability and clarity.

Onward to healing and good health!

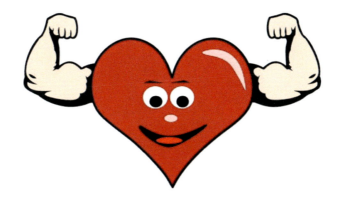

Oriental Medicine

In the early 1970s the media increased its focus on life inside China. The American public was introduced to China's massive health care system which used many ancient, yet effective medical methods. It was acupuncture that seemed to catch America's attention most of all. It was not the only part of traditional Oriental Medicine, nor was it even the single most used part of that system. Acupuncture was simply best suited to our very visual media.

Time and *Newsweek* quickly realized that pictures of acupuncture attracted attention. Because of this media emphasis on acupuncture, those who practiced Oriental Medicine in the United States came to be called "acupuncturists," even though they were trained in a much larger context, and usually did other traditional therapies in addition to acupuncture. Acupuncture is part of that rich tradition of Oriental Medicine which uses many therapeutic approaches, unified by extensive philosophical and diagnostic understandings.

In understanding these philosophical and diagnostic understandings, let us take a look at the importation of Oriental Medicine to the United States. In order to teach Oriental Medicine to Americans, the classical Chinese texts were translated into English. Of course, we know that in all walks of life there is always something lost in translation.

As an example, let us take the basic term in Chinese for Liver. The word in Chinese for Liver is "Gan." When a Doctor of Oriental Medicine is using the word Gan, there is much more understood by that word than the mere physical organ that resides under the right rib cage. This word also describes the emotions that are associated with Gan, such as anger, resentment, frustration, depression, emotional repression, stubbornness, irrationality, aggression, and indecisiveness.

Also implicit in the word Gan is the knowledge that the Gan nourishes the tendons and ligaments in the body. The Gan is responsible for our capacity for planning. The Gan is also responsible for nourishing the eyes. The Gan is responsible for headaches that manifest in the top of the head. The Gan is responsible for problems that seem to arise between 1:00 a.m. and 3:00 a.m. The Gan is responsible for ailments that seem to arise in the Spring. The Gan is responsible for ailments that can be traced along the external and internal acupuncture meridians from the big toe, to the inner leg to surround the genitals, connect with the Gall Bladder, and continuing up to surround the breasts. The nickname in Oriental Medicine for Gan is *The General*, because the Gan is responsible for the smooth flowing function of everything in the body, mind, emotions, and spirit. To carry this further, there is a two-way street, where the Gan can affect all of these aspects of our humanness, and the aspects of our humanness can affect the Gan.

We can see the richness of this term. When the translators of the classics translated this word, Gan into English, the closest that we can get to it is Liver, thereby losing the richness of the word. When the practitioner of Oriental Medicine is talking about the Liver to his or her patients or other English speaking people he or she is using the term Liver, but is thinking Gan.

From this perspective we need to define the larger

rubric of Oriental Medicine. Listed in their order of efficacy, these are the nine traditional branches of Oriental Medicine:

1. Meditation
2. Dietetics
3. Herbs
4. Movement (Tai Chi/Qi Gong)
5. Acupuncture
6. Massage
7. Sexual Practices
8. Geomancy (Feng Shui)
9. Numerology

Each of these alone would be a topic for lifetime study, but the proficient doctor of Oriental Medicine (OM) has at least a working knowledge of all of these branches.

Although OM derived from Taoist, Buddhist, and Confucian lineage, it was undoubtedly most influenced by its Taoist roots.

The Taoists were an interesting group. One group was comprised of the disenchanted philosophers of the Warring States (about 200 AD to 200 BC), who felt that the chaos in the world could not be addressed directly. They felt it pointless to try to initiate reform, and so decided to split apart from society and align themselves with nature. Because they were, however, more citified and more literary, they took with them to the mountains many of their literary traditions, i.e., science, divination, astronomy, and astrology.

When they got to the mountains, they met and interacted with the native shamanic people, who grew up there studying herbs, watching the celestial patterns, studying animals, digging for minerals, and developing a grassroots science based on empirical evidence. As these diverse groups began to commingle, the more literary recorded some of the history, tradition and practices of the rural shamanic people. Together, they began to follow the way of nature.

The Taoists were, in essence, Qi worshippers. They spent much of their time cultivating and accumulating Qi. They were obsessed with long life. However, this was not merely for the venal purpose of reaching any chronological milestone. The Taoists felt that if one lived a long time, then that would allow a person more time to do the spiritual practices which would accumulate and refine their Qi. They would then be better able to deal with, and move on to the next level of experience after they, as spiritual beings, had finished having their human experience. Therefore, because the first requisite of a long life is a healthy life, most medical practices derived from this Taoist tradition. This concept of Qi is one which bears some explanation, since it is foreign to most westerners.

Here it is helpful to bring our attention to the ultimate in human experience—death. Let us imagine a situation in which we are with someone who is near death. Now the person is alive and two seconds later the person is dead. What has changed? The blood is still there. The hormones are still there. The neurotransmitters are still there. The antibodies are still there. All the chemicals that we have in life are still there. What has changed is that there is no more Life Force (Qi) which is continuing to make the life-fostering chemical changes do what they have done since birth. The only chemical changes happening from death onward are geared to turn us into dust. This Life-Force (Qi-Energy) courses through our bodies in prescribed pathways and its unimpeded flow determines our health or lack thereof.

We derive our Vital Force (Qi) from three primary sources. The first source is from our parents. This is called Prenatal Qi. This is fixed in the amount that we receive based upon the health of our parents. We use this Qi in our transition through our various life stages from infancy to childhood to adolescence to adulthood to old age. If our Prenatal is deficient right from the get-go, then we age faster and are plagued with more health problems throughout life than someone who has greater Prenatal Qi. As Prenatal Qi is used up we age and move closer to our final curtain. However, we can delay the ultimate by conserving the Prenatal Qi as much as possible by conservation practices and living a healthy life style.

Another source of our Vital Force (Qi) is the food and drink that we consume. Processed, adulterated, fractionated foods have no life giving ability and drain our Vital Force (Qi). We use food and drink to replenish the energy that we have used up from our daily activities. When we use up more energy than we are able to replenish with food and drink, then we dip into our Prenatal Qi in order to maintain function. This ages us faster.

The other place we get energy is from the air that we breathe. Practicing breathing exercises on a regular basis helps us to increase our Qi.

The above lays a basis for a brief discussion of the nine major branches of Traditional Chinese Medicine (TCM).

Meditation

Meditation is first in importance because it is the most fundamental way to gather energy to yourself.

Meditation gathers in energy with a minimum outflow of energy. Meditation is the most direct route to making contact with the Vital Force, the Qi; that which is the only thing that heals us and keeps us alive. The connection with and the accumulation and nurturing of this energy is the only thing that allows us to heal ourselves and others. The doctor just sends the bill.

Dietetics

In dietetics it is important to know whether a food is *building* or *cleansing*. The protein foods are building foods, whereas fruits are cleansing foods. Grains are rather neutral, so they act as a good base from which to start. Cooking basically adds Qi to your food and makes them more digestible. The Chinese method of stir-fry preparation accomplishes this goal without destroying the important enzymes needed to digest that particular food which are part and parcel of that food.

Raw foods have reached acclaim in the United States because the traditional American diet can be binding and constricting. Raw foods open one up. However, once opened up, this type of diet will become depleting.

Herbs

The more *de-tuned* a person is to the environment, the more intense a treatment is needed. Herbs generally come after dietetics, which is a necessary foundation for any herbal work. With poor dietetics, herbs will not have optimum effect, or only will give temporary relief. Poor diet in and of itself can become an OBSTACLE TO CURE.

About 80% of the western herbal books on the market are about folk medicine. They will indicate, for example, 46 herbs for headache, and 25 herbs for upset stomach. How do you pick and choose? One headache or stomachache is not the same as another headache or stomachache.

It is a fallacy to believe that because herbs are natural, they are easy to use and can cause no harm. For example, many herbs have cooling or warming qualities. It would generally not be appropriate to give herbs which would be "cooling" to someone who is shivering. The magic word in the last sentence is *generally*. Depending on the complex of symptoms and signs that go together to make the person, all rules are merely guidelines which may be used and altered with the particular case.

Movement (Tai Chi/Qi Gong)

There are two broad categories of movement: therapeutic movement and martial movement, and they both have some common aspects. Among the therapeutic movements are hundreds of Taoist meditative, therapeutic movements, such as Qi Gong.

One system of Qi Gong is the Five Animal Frolics. These exercises by Hua To, considered by many as China's most famous physician, are based on the movements of the bear, deer, crane, monkey and tiger. Their function is to open up the energy channels. To translate, Qi Gong means to do "energy work." Qi is the life energy, and Gong means actually to do hard work over a period of time.

The most popular system of therapeutic movement in the US is Tai Chi. Tai Chi is a way of making direct contact with the Qi, and experiencing the flow of that Qi throughout the energy channels. When one is practiced at experiencing the flow of Qi, one can also feel the blockages in the flow and can then direct the Qi to push through that blockage. Blocked Qi equals sickness and death; free flowing Qi equals health and life. There is no better form of therapy for those having balance problems than Tai Chi.

Acupuncture

With acupuncture, the flow and balance of Qi are affected by the insertion of fine shafts of steel into appropriate points on the body. We think of it as almost like a key which opens up the gate and allows the energy to flow the way it is supposed to.

Herbal medicine is generally better for building the patient, and acupuncture is generally better for clearing energetic blockages. Acupuncture is, however, not the mere insertion of needles into the correct locations. There is also a subtle transference of energy that is happening in the treatment session. A Chinese saying captures this well: "When your heart is pure, the gods ride on the end of the needle and every point is an acupuncture point." Intention is even more important than location. (Do you want someone sticking needles into you who has just had a fight with their significant other?)

There is a disturbing trend in the allopathic medical community to see acupuncture as a mere modality which can be mastered in a couple hundred hours. Acupuncture, taken outside the context of Oriental Medicine, is ineffective and potentially dangerous.

It is not possible to look up a point prescription in a textbook for back pain, use those points, and expect that any sizable percentage of those suffering from back pain will receive any relief. Practitioners of OM do not treat back pain. They treat people who have back pain. This is an important distinction.

Back pain is only one component of a person. That back pain will express itself within the matrix of that person's personality and underlying energetic disorder.

For instance, one person's back pain may be made worse with movement, heat, or at night. She or he may have a boisterous personality with a tendency to anger. Another person may have back pain which will be worse while the person is staying still, cold, or during the day. That person may have a tendency to feel low energetically.

This first person would fit into a pattern of disharmony in Oriental Medicine known as deficiency of liver Qi, or wood overacting on the water element. The second would fit into a pattern of disharmony in OM known as deficient kidney Qi. Each of these people with low back pain is going to need a completely different method of treatment using acupuncture and/or moxibustion.

Acupuncture needs to be used and understood in its context as a part of OM, and not just as a modality to be used cookbook style. Those teaching abbreviated courses to allied health professionals do a great disservice to the profession of OM, to themselves, and to patients. Patients who go to those who are trained via abbreviated courses don't get results. They then erroneously decide that acupuncture doesn't work, and therefore suffer needlessly.

Massage-Bodywork

We all have certain blockages in our body with which we, ourselves, cannot deal directly because we are causing them in the first place. To have someone get in there is extremely important because we cannot always relieve our own imbalances (an arrogant assumption). The same caveat would hold here as with acupuncture. The intention of the massage therapist needs to be totally here and now and with the patient, and not on the vagaries of their own life. Again, this is because it is not merely a process of moving body tissues around. There is also a subtle transference of energy between the massage therapist and the patient.

Sexual Practices

This was originally the secret of the emperors who might have as many as 50 wives. One can only imagine how depleting those would become for anyone. For men, the emphasis was on conserving their "Jing," which can be best translated as sperm, as too many ejaculations would be a serious drain on a man's Vital Force. For women, the emphasis was on creating good circulation for the movement of fluids and blood. Sex was used by the Taoists as a way of attaining higher levels of spirituality, much in the way of the Indian Tantric tradition. It was a way of transferring, building, sharing and balancing one's energy with one's partner's energy, and vice versa.

Geomancy (Feng Shui)

This comes from the Chinese words "Feng Shui," which means wind and water. Feng Shui is the art of wind and water. The implication is that wind and water are always moving and changing. The very word conjures up the idea of observing Qi in motion.

This might come into play when we have tried everything and nothing seems to be working. Here the OM practitioner might want to go to the home of the patient and see if there are any environmental disturbances which could be changed.

For instance, someone who lives at the center of the

top of a "T" formed by two perpendicular streets would be living in a configuration called the Arrows of Death. This is a position in which your house is constantly and directly bombarded with Qi. Actually, common sense would tell you that you do not want to be living in this house. At night, the headlights of cars driving up the street would hit your house at all hours.

Interestingly, the Chinese see money as the consolidation of Qi, so this configuration would actually be a good position for a business. For a residence, however, it is not so good. You will find people who live in this configuration are generally poor in health, have difficulties financially, and difficulties in relationships on many different levels.

The good news is that it is fixable. In order to ameliorate the effects of this constant bombardment of Qi, you would do something, such as planting bushes in front of the house to absorb the excess Qi, or building a pond in front of the house with a winding pathway to the front door. We have all been in places where we just feel "funny." We get a contracted feeling every time we are in that place. When we live in that place and have to constantly contract many times a day, this unbalances us energetically. Ultimately, it will manifest on a physical level, but no lab test will show the root of the pathology. This is the realm in which Feng Shui acts, and it can be a powerful healer in the hands of someone knowledgeable in its use.

Numerology-Divination

For those situations which elude the rational mind, where you have done all of the correct treatments with no results, there may be another factor. This is where you would resort to divination, and do a psychic reading, or read a five element palm, or consult the I Ching. This is certainly not the optimum treatment modality, but it beats telling the patient, "You have to learn to live with it," or "There is nothing that can be done for you."

• • •

I hope you are left with the impression that OM is a comprehensive medical system which must be used from its own perspective, and not judged from the perspective of the western model. All systems of medicine have their rightful place, and when practiced by the well-trained doctor, the patient gets the best of all worlds.

Letters from the Heart

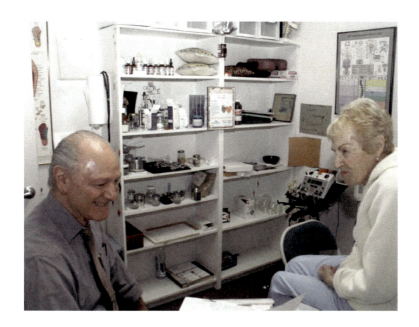

Working with children

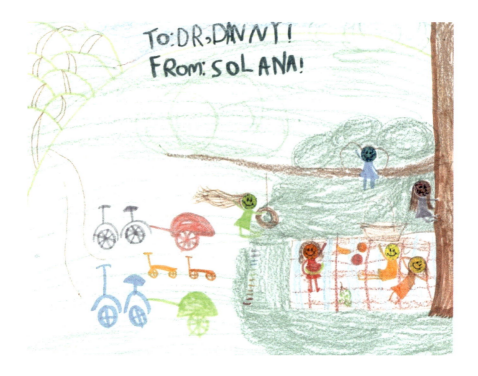

I decided to place this section first because the healing children receive allows them to thrive for a lifetime instead of spending years battling seemingly intractable problems.

We don't receive many testimonials from children, so I thought to relate my experience with my younger patients. The drawings are some of my prized possessions because they are from the heart and unfiltered.

An interesting thing happened when we changed the name of the practice from the Acupuncture Center of Vero Beach to the Alternative Medicine Family Care Center. The services that we provided did not change, only the name. Unexpectedly we began seeing children become patients—a lot of them. How to explain this? Perhaps a child might not be not keen going to the Acu**PUNCTURE** Center.

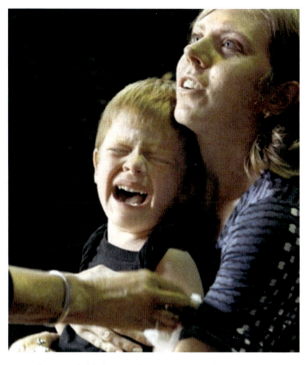

I love treating children because they make me look so good. They get better quickly, possibly because they haven't had much time to develop the severe pathologies of their adult counterparts.

I recall one 4 year-old boy who was having an earache. His mother wanted to take him to the emergency room. He screamed his protestation, "No, I don't want to go to the hospital. I want to go to Dr. Danny!" Children respond very well to homeopathic medicine, and the remedies have a sweet taste, so kids are eager to take them. Thank you Samuel Hahnemann.

My youngest patient was seven weeks old. This poor baby was allergic to mom's milk. It doesn't get any more basic than that. I treated the baby using the Natural Allergy Elimination Technique one time. Mom was then able to nurse her baby without vomiting the milk. That one treatment to eliminate the allergy to mom's milk changed that baby's life forever.

A mom called the office and related that she had just eaten a peanut butter sandwich, after which she kissed her son who then went into anaphylactic shock. She injected him with an Epi-Pen (epinephrine injection) and rushed him to the hospital. I told her to bring him in and to bring the peanut butter too. I put the peanut butter into a vial, tested him, and treated him that day. I told mom to bring him back the next day so that I could test him again to make sure that the treatment worked. He tested fine with the peanut butter. I sent my assistant across the street to get a Reese's Peanut Butter Cup. She brought it back. We gave it to the boy. He ate the peanut butter cup. No reaction! The way things ought to be.

Another mom brought her daughter to see me. She had been given a diagnosis of ADHD. She was not able to do school work. We worked to clear a few allergies, but the most profound change happened when I convinced her to change her diet and stop eating the sugary breakfasts. Her mom called and thanked me for giving her child back to her.

Another 4 year-old boy had been constipated for two years. It had reached the point where he actually had to go to the hospital and have the stools physically extracted. It was about to reach that point again. Over the course of two years, mom had tried everything to help her son—herbs, laxatives, medications. Nothing worked. When I see someone, I always try to learn that "Not Been Well Since" moment. I asked her a question that no one had ever asked. "What was happening two years ago when it all began?" She said, "He was molested by his step brother." My first thought was it would be futile to address this with herbs and acupuncture. Instead I gave him a dose of a homeopathic medicine only once. Well, mom called me back three days later saying he was on the toilet, and bragging to mom about being able to go to the bathroom.☺ I still get chills when I think about that kid.

These are only a few of many such stories. Of course, it's not only the parents who are thrilled and grateful, but the children as well, who often express such things through pictures. After all, a picture is worth a thousand words.

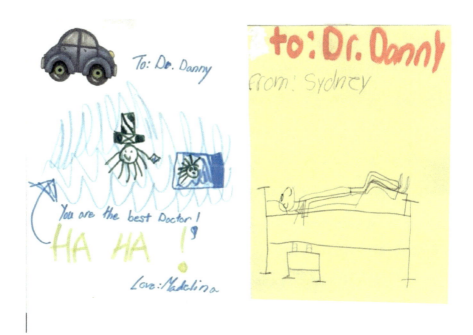

Acupuncture

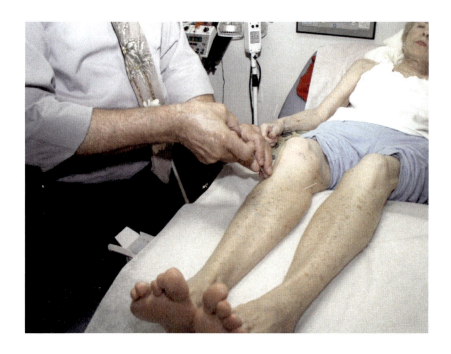

To be honest, I did not know if acupuncture would be of any help.

When I first visited you I was impressed by your gentle confidence and respect for me. My first treatment was not painful, and I forgot about it until several days later. I had been given instructions to do hand movement exercises after surgery. One morning upon waking, I noticed my fingers and hand were not swollen! The acupuncture had started working!

You continued to work patiently with me, as I progressed in a most positive direction.

I hope others read of my experience so they realize how acupuncture can help them.

And to you Dr. Danny Quaranto, I thank you for

your caring and understanding. Your friend.

• • •

Dear Dr. Quaranto,

I will forever be grateful for your dedicated treatment of my ailments from my car accident. It was fortunate that I chose you to introduce me to acupuncture and administer to my needs.

Thank you for changing my life for the better. Sincerely PS I miss you already!

• • •

To whom it may concern,

After spending considerable time and money with doctors with little or no satisfaction, I decided to go to The Acupuncture Center of Vero Beach.

I was so impressed with the benefits from my treatment. I now walk well, the headaches are gone, and the dizziness is in control.

I hope this letter will give confidence to anyone to go for treatment. Sincerely.

• • •

Dear Danny,

Many, many thanks for the acupuncture therapy you gave me. It works! More than that, I appreciate your kindness and encouragement to help myself. I am trying the Tai Chi; it also helps, and has become easier now.

As soon as possible, I hope to continue the acupuncture once a month, if you will accept me.

Usually my coping skills are fine. Sometimes I run out of "Cope," but not Hope. Thank you from my heart!

• • •

Dear Dr. Dan,

I've been meaning to write you for weeks since my return to Ottawa, to tell you how the acupuncture treatments relieved my painful back after my fall, just before I left for Florida last year. In addition, my energy level has increased tremendously along with a significant decrease in angina distress.

If I were coming to Vero this winter, you would surely find me in your office again because of my trouble with chronic bronchitis, pneumonia, and respiratory allergies. I really must find an acupuncture physician here in Ottawa to control my weak respiratory system.

Wishing you continued success in your excellent service, and helping people overcome pain and strengthen their energy fields.

• • •

(This is a letter to a congressman that references treatment by Dr. Quaranto.)

H.R. 2588, The Federal Acupuncture Act, now pending before the House, is of great significance.

I have suffered for many years from an immune system disease diagnosed at one time as Systemic Lupus Erythematosus, another time as Lupus Arthritis, another time as degenerative joint disease, another time as vascular disease of undetermined etiology, and others.

I have been treated by rheumatologists, internists, neurologists, physical therapists, and so on. I have taken many anti-inflammatory drugs, both steroidal and non-steroidal, for fifteen years, with variable success—but never without pain and discomfort to my legs, particularly my knees, and back pain so serious I've had surgery twice. I could go on about my troubles, but you don't need to hear all that. What I hope will get your attention and your support for H.R.2588.

My son-in-law, Donald xxxx, M.D., has used acupuncture when appropriate for some twenty years. He recommended that I try it. Dr. Danny Quaranto has treated me here in Vero Beach with what I can describe as almost miraculous results. The pain I had endured for so long is GONE!!!

Dr. Quaranto does not claim that this improvement is permanent or that my troubles are over. But for me, this experience testifies impressively to the efficacy of acupuncture.

Furthermore, recent recognition that alternative medical disciplines provide real value to healthcare in Western cultures is noteworthy. I am absolutely positive that all of American healthcare will benefit when—not if— acupuncture is recognized and accepted by our medical authorities and by the people of our country. Congress can hasten this time if it passes H.R 2588. I ask that you do everything in your power to advance the progress and the passage of this legislation.

Thank you for your attention.

• • •

Wish I could get in touch with the whole world

of afflicted people, whether they have a major or minor discomfort, to tell them of the wonderful results I've obtained from you through acupuncture.

Allergies

Natural Allergy Elimination Technique

To whom it may concern,

Last year I was treated by Dr. Danny Quaranto for a long-standing allergy to strawberries. I would break out with hives followed by intense itching.

After one treatment using his Natural Allergy Elimination Technique I was able to eat strawberries again with no allergic response. In fact, one day after the treatment I had the opportunity to eat strawberries and did so with no adverse effects. This treatment is still working well after one year.

• • •

My medical history regarding allergies is one of unsatisfactory relief and wasted dollars. I have had scratch testing followed by years of allergy injections, beginning at age eighteen; several years at a clinic in Cocoa Beach with little progress; and years of taking over-the-counter remedies which only mask and suppress symptoms rather than alleviate them. These years of treatment cost me an estimated $23,000.

Dr. Quaranto has treated me for a number of allergens, including chocolate, cats, pollen, orange blossoms, vegetables, caffeine, eggs, and molds. As a result of the allergy elimination I feel wonderful throughout the winter—a new experience for me. I am able to eat any food and feel great.

In addition, my asthma condition is gone and I have an enhanced sense of health and vitality.

Dr. Quaranto uses a combination of care modalities from acupuncture to homeopathy and herbs. I believe these solutions, together with his caring rapport and careful listening so he *hears* his patients, were crucial factors in my ability to heal and become virtually allergy-free.

• • •

Dear Dr. Quaranto,

As a result of your care I no longer suffer from allergies that impacted my health, some being life-long.

Dr. Quaranto treated me for celery allergy. I was previously unable to eat celery without sneezing and congestion for several hours. I was not able to even be in the house when my husband juiced celery. After a single treatment I eat celery as often and as much as I want without any symptoms.

He treated my allergy to dairy and calcium as well. Certain milk products had caused indigestion, often with sacroiliac and neck pain. Both required frequent chiropractic adjustments. Since completing treatment, I no longer have indigestion because of milk products, and seldom do I have neck or back pain. I now see my chiropractor only quarterly. She is amazed and remarked that whatever I am doing, keep it up. I told her I'd already done it!

Another allergy treated was mold and dust. The results have also been astounding. I actually breathe through my nose while sleeping for the first time I can remember. I do housework and make beds without sneezing. Dust is no longer a problem.

Also treated were allergies to sugar and grains, which substantially improved my quality of life. I no longer experience headaches, nausea, and low blood sugar after eating sugar; and I no longer have digestive problems when I eat products containing oat bran.

I plan to continue treatment until all my allergies are eliminated. I have tried many traditional treatments, including allergy shots, elimination-rotation diets, cortisone shots, Prednisone, etc. Throughout my life this is the only thing that has worked for me.

My allergies are well documented from multiple medical tests. My family allergist has become interested in the technique and is excited about retesting me at the conclusion of my treatment to convince himself that it works. Obviously, I'm already convinced!

So, thank you, Danny, for such an excellent treatment. You are offering an invaluable service that everyone should know about!

Alternative medicine

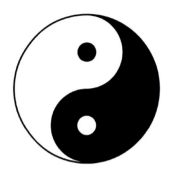

To Whom It May Concern,

Before my first visit to Danny Quaranto one year ago, I had suffered from migraine headaches more than ten years, had sinus surgery twice, underwent all kinds of diagnostic procedures, and had been on drugs ranging from over the counter pain relief to massive doses of antibiotics to narcotics. I had been to all types of medical doctors and none could offer lasting relief. It seemed these so-called medical doctors could only offer help with a prescription pad, treating the symptoms rather than finding a cure.

My insurance company paid more than $60,000 to these "medical" doctors, labs, and pharmacies. I of course had the expense of not only the premiums but also the deductibles, non-covered, and co-pays, plus what I spent at the pharmacy myself. More important than the wasted money was the damage to my body, both physically and emotionally.

By the time a friend mentioned acupuncture and Danny Quaranto, I was frustrated with the medical profession and willing to try anything. I had almost resigned myself living in pain for the rest of my life.

My first visit with Dr. Dan was the beginning of a

new and improved life for myself, as well as my family. Yes, they also suffered with me all those years. Dr. Dan was confident he could relieve my pain, and was able to explain the problem in basic English. My body was reacting badly to certain foods as well as environmental toxins. Dr. Dan told me that my body was not properly assimilating foods thereby causing the reactions. He felt that with acupuncture he could put my body back in proper balance.

The night of the first visit provided encouragement I had not before felt. Each subsequent visit reinforced it as I felt better and better. I could eat foods and be places that before would have caused an instant migraine. Three months and $1,500 later (the best money I ever spent) I became, and remain, a new, drug-free person thanks to Dr. Dan.

My insurance does not cover acupuncture; most companies don't. If they really cared to cut costs and improve health, as they claim, why don't they reconsider? It doesn't take a genius to know spending $1,500 versus $60,000 says it all. Additionally, if the medical profession really wanted to make people well, they would consider referring some of their patients to an acupuncture physician. Acupuncture has been around for a thousand years or so. I don't ever remember hearing a recall for that treatment.

If I sound pleased with Dr. Dan and not so pleased with members of the so-called medical profession, then you have read and understood this letter as it was intended. Dr. Dan *did* deliver to me a better life thanks to his talent and real caring of the individuals he treats.

As I said in the beginning, I was referred by a friend, and have since, and will continue to refer people to him. I trust him totally.

Arthritis

To whom it may concern,

I searched for alternative healthcare when I developed arthritis in my left hip and right knee. I walked with a cane with considerable pain. After six acupuncture treatments from Dr. Quaranto, I am happy to say I no longer need my cane. And I am bowling and walking again. Dr. Quaranto treated me for high blood pressure and brought the pressure down 40 points in a week with the aid of Chinese herbs.

I would recommend when going for acupuncture, do so with a positive attitude. It will help with the treatments.

• • •

I'm writing this so that you can place it in your testimonials book so if others have a problem like mine they can feel comfortable coming to you for treatment.

I started to get severe pain below the left and right shoulders and above my right ear causing severe headaches lasting 8-10 hours. A chiropractor took x-rays and diagnosed me with arthritis. I took 8-10 treatments—no results. I decided to see an orthopedic doctor for a second opinion; he took more x-rays, same diagnosis. He advised me to take physical therapy treatments. I took 10-12 treatments; the pain was still severe and I was getting depressed and upset by the medical bills.

Then I met a patient from Alternative Medicine

Family Care Center who recommended that I try acupuncture. I took four treatments and the pain gradually eased up with no more headaches, which had been severe. I started to feel *much* better; I felt like a new person.

I sincerely recommend patients with arthritis problems to contact Alternative Medicine Family Care Center of Vero Beach. I am sure you too will get results.

When you take treatments from Danny Quaranto, you will find him to be sincere and understanding. It's a pleasure to have someone listen so well and caringly. Great asset to the arthritis patient.

• • •

Dear Danny,

I wish I could get in touch with the whole world of afflicted people, whether it be a major or minor discomfort, to tell them of the wonderful results from your acupuncture.

As you know, when I first came to you I was unable to walk across the room without the aid of a cane or hanging onto the furniture. This resulted from a severe arthritic condition, in particular, a hip replacement that was not working well. Nothing I did would help. I was going downhill and seemed destined to depend on painkillers for the rest of my life.

I don't know whether it was the needles or the other medication, or both, but to me it was miraculous. Since the short six or eight visits to you, I have not once used my cane and am relatively free of pain most of the time. I enjoy a feeling of general well-being all the time.

I recommend acupuncture to anyone.

Cancer

In 2002 I was diagnosed with stage four metastatic melanoma. I was also the sole parent to a 3-year-old girl. To make matters worse, the surgeon cut the melanoma so the risk of cancer seeding was present. I was given a few months to live by all the doctors I saw, both locally and those in the big research centers of Florida.

They offered only one treatment option—at $70,000! and I was uninsured. They admitted it wouldn't really increase my chances of survival. One doctor, however, did give me a prescription with instructions "to take it all when things get bad."

A friend then referred me to Doctor Danny who gave me a homeopathic medicine that I took for a few months. When I went to the oncologist after three months they did more images. They showed that the nodules around my neck were clear! Wow! The oncologists were baffled. I remain free from cancer to this day, with PET scans in 2008 and 2012 showing clear.

Doctor Danny helped a miracle happen with my cancer.

Homeopathy

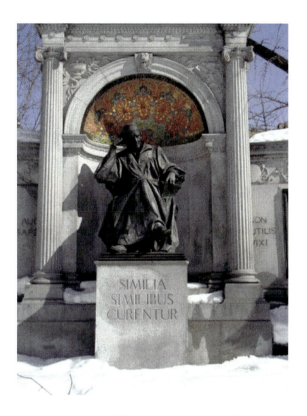

Samuel Hahnemann, MD

From Dr. Danny:

The Hahnemann Monument in Washington, D.C. is the only monument of its type in Washington dedicated to a foreign physician. This is a man who in the context of his one life conceived, developed, and perfected a complete medical system.

Chinese medicine has been a continual growth process built upon the shoulders of 5,000 years of researchers. By contrast, conventional medicine has had a continual growth only since Hippocrates 2,000 years ago.

Hahnemann did it all while under the constant vilification of the conventional medical establishment, whose true motivation was to protect its own little rice bowl.

If I had one person in history at whose feet I would sit and soak up his or her wisdom, it would not be Sun Si Miao or Hua To, it would be Samuel Hahnemann.

Truly every homeopath in the world will claim pon experiencing the power of homeopathic medicine on their patients that, "All Praise Goes to Hahnemann." Indeed his epitaph rings true, more than two hundred years after his death. "I have not lived in vain." How many of us would live, just to be able to claim that at the end. Homeopathy is the place I go when I'm looking for a miracle.

• • •

Dear Danny!

A note to let you know the results of the vaccination emergency ordeal. The baby suffered a cerebral hemorrhage the size of a golf ball along with seizures. All within three days of his vaccinations. The hospital doctors denied it was vaccine damage, but the symptoms say otherwise.

Within 30 minutes of orally taking the (homeopathic) remedy, this 3½ month-old baby fell peacefully asleep. Before the remedy he had symptoms of extreme irritability, vomiting, restlessness, sleeplessness, no desire for breast milk, loud, whiny crying—and much more. This went on for days immediately after the vaccinations.

I investigated and discovered that there are more than 1000 reports each month from parents and doctors, indicating many acute and chronic symptoms are related to vaccines. It's disgusting how this government has mandatory vaccine laws with so many deaths and brain-damaged children directly related to this problem.

The good thing is that we have homeopathy. We couldn't save even one baby's life without it, as I was able to do. The doctor gave him three options: brain surgery, brain damage, or death! One small (homeopathy) pellet and a child lives. How amazing is that! The follow-up CAT scan and x-ray showed no signs of a hemorrhage!

I share this with you because only a homeopath would understand.

Thanks again Dr. Danny. With love.

• • •

Dear Danny,

Thank you so much for the excellent homeopathy course. I thoroughly enjoyed it and the company of my classmates!

Your knowledge is tremendous, as is your dedication to healing. My Andrew Lockie book arrived in the mail yesterday. I sat in the garage and started reading it. It's addictive, and it keeps my mind off other stuff! Thanks Danny.

• • •

The homeopathic drops have worked so well, especially Envirox2 Asthma. I now eat pasta every day, and gelato!

• • •

Hi Dr. Danny,

My knee feels so much better. It is a little sore from the treatment yesterday but I didn't have to use anything to ease it. After many years of putting up with aches and pains, this seems too good to be true. But then again so is homeopathy. The one dose I took in the office seemed to do the trick for my bladder problem.

As I get ready to move from Florida, I am thinking how lucky I was to find you when I lived here. My search for a perfect health doctor ended with you. I have been to many natural health practitioners and tried everything. Acupuncture helped at times, but it wasn't complete. I also tried herbs, Reiki, chiropractic--you name it. I have little faith in allopathic doctors and abhor taking meds. I was always looking for answers myself, so in my search I tried many things and many paths. I was always interested in natural cures and herbs as a way of letting my body heal without the harsh medicines. I guess that is why I like homeopathy so much.

The classes I took with you were most interesting. I mentioned them to my sister and she may sign up for next year's class. She is also interested in homeopathic remedies and I know she would benefit from taking your class. Perhaps she will discover what a great person you are as I did. I know her funds are limited because she is a widow and doesn't have a large income, but the cost doesn't seem so great in the end. My cure has been gentle and I feel so much better.

Thank you from the bottom of my heart. Have a good summer.

Prolotherapy

Regenerative Injection Therapy

Danny,

You are truly amazing!

Thank you so much for coming in on Saturday to treat my Achilles. I walked two miles on Saturday and Sunday and feel great! I left on my road trip adventure early this morning feeling energized. I would not be traveling today had you not helped me on Saturday. I am so grateful!

A friend of mine is going to be a new patient of yours in October.

I read most of your book last evening. Truly inspiring!!! I'm going to send copies to my daughters. Many thanks.

See you in October...unless I fall in love. ☺ Love and light to you.

A word from the author about Prolotherapy.

Prolotherapy is an injection therapy which has a 60 year history. It is the opposite of a steroid injection. In fact, the active ingredient injected is Dextrose, also known as sugar. The amount used is minimal, so it is quite safe to use, even for diabetics.

Why does it work? It works because it utilizes the body's own natural inflammatory response to assist in the healing of injured ligaments and tendons. The mild inflammatory response that results from the injection stimulates your body to bring chondroblasts, fibroblasts, collagen, and elastin—substances that comprise connective tissue—to the affected area that builds new tissue and tightens lax ligaments.

Next time you have a chicken dinner look at the tendons and ligaments. They are white or clear. This indicates there is little blood supply to those tissues. When they become injured they do not heal very well, if at all, and we get recurrent injury to that same area. Prolotherapy is a method of increasing circulation to the area so the body can heal itself. No drugs are used.

Pain Relief

Dear Dr. Danny,

 I would like to start by saying *thank you*. I currently feel better than I have in years. Meeting you has been a life-changing experience. I appreciate your patience and willingness to listen and find the root cause of the issues presented to you. You are the first medical professional who I felt actually listened to my problems and truthfully who I felt actually listened to my problems and truthfully wanted to help me. I had grown accustomed to having my ailments brushed aside and being written a prescription to "fix" it.

 Upon arriving home in West Virginia, I have noticed I no longer have congestion and sinus issues I once dealt with and assumed was normal. Since beginning treatments, I have not suffered from any migraines. I can feel that I am becoming more rational calm, and confident. I am not living in a constant state of fear and worry and that itself is a true blessing. I am proud to say that I am driving more and will be starting a new job next week

 For the first time that I can remember I am excited for the future and what it might bring. Again, thank you for all that you have done for me. I look forward to seeing you in December.

Dear Dr. Quaranto,

 Your acupuncture treatments have enabled me to lead a normal life, one without pain and limitations. I had suffered since 1985 from whiplash from an auto accident. I had been in constant neck pain, along with headaches and fatigue. I am feeling energetic again and now work in the yard without pain and discomfort.

Acupuncture may not be for everyone, but it definitely helped me.

• • •

Dear Ms. Rodham Clinton:

Please convince the F.D.A. to upgrade Acupuncture's experimental status to *approved*, and include Acupuncture in the National Healthcare Initiative.

I speak from personal experience. My shoulder had suffered a fractured clavicle and two separations, resulting in enough damage to the muscle cuff and persistent excruciating chronic pain that my orthopedic surgeon said surgery was the only solution.

However, while on vacation, I visited the Acupuncture Center of Vero Beach, Florida, in a desperate attempt to obtain some relief. After only four weeks, two visits per week, the pain was gone!

Some will doubtlessly claim coincidence, or the warm climate made the difference. Well, I hope everyone that has suffered so miserably for twelve long years gets the same relief in only four short weeks.

I hope you and the National Healthcare Initiative make Acupuncture a viable alternative treatment program.

• • •

Dear Dr. Quaranto,

I wish to thank you for your concern for my

daughter. I feared for her life several months ago. I mean this literally. She was in such constant pain and so desperate. Improvement since being treated by you has been a relief to us both!

Please don't be discouraged if she is not responding as you would like. She may never be "normal" as we see it, but you are controlling the severity of her pain, and most importantly, have given her hope, hope that she had almost lost.

Thanks also for your concern for me. We need more doctors like you!

• • •

Dear Dr. Danny,

The greatest thing I ever did was call your office a couple of years ago when my shoulder was giving me so much pain! Your acupuncture treatments cured it, diverted it, disguised it, or whatever—but it's gone!!

I'm spreading the word.

• • •

Hi Doc!

Thanks for replying.☺ Yesterday's text was nice. I can't claim complete removal of pain—yet, but I feel so different somewhere inside.

Yesterday I came in miserable, all my pain areas kickin', and when I left my mind didn't seem to immediately find them to focus on again. I had K take me directly to the Ocean, the one place I can truly think. Or not think most of the time. I would love to call it meditation, but I must struggle very hard to push out negative thoughts, mostly stressors.

And the cleansing from the hurricane reminded me

of what I've begun to do by coming to your office. But we could only stay a few moments. And I could only *fight it*—I guess that would be the term—for a few more hours. Today's another day. ☺

• • •

Sorry about the rambling email. My friends say I talk enough for eight people. Even K said, "Keep it short, Doc's a busy guy."

Not only did I not get to see you for a few weeks, my therapist left the state for a month during the storms and isn't scheduled back till early next week. But I think I faired okay considering how I may have handled the storm, etc. a year back.

Well, I'll let you get back to your good work and look forward to three days a week with you. Here's to safe drivers and motorcycle helmets allowed in cars!

Thanks for your time.

• • •

Your acupuncture treatment greatly relieved the pain in my lower back and wrist. The procedure instantly stopped my back spasms. It also improved the strength of my wrists.

• • •

Dear Danny,

I just wanted to thank you for relieving the pain in my arm and getting it mobile. I've told my friends that acupuncture is worth trying. It certainly worked for me! Sincerely.

Smoking

Dr. Quaranto,

I am most grateful for the experience of your program that enabled me to quit smoking. I am excited to have reached my goal. As a non-smoker, I am looking forward to many more health goals. Your program and your help will have a lasting effect. Thank you.

I'd like also to thank Angela whose positive and helpful personality was a pleasure. Much happiness and appreciation.

• • •

Dear Dr. Quaranto,

I believe in acupuncture. I had medical shots for neck pains over the past three years. However, the relief didn't last. But after acupuncture I now feel more comfortable.

You also stopped my smoking, much to my husband's delight. In the fall, I intend to return for more acupuncture treatments to regain my sense of smell. Gratefully.

Surgery

In deciding what to do, I trusted you. I needed an authority outside myself. I thank you for your time, patience, presence, and kindness.

It kinda went like: if you thought it was okay to have surgery, maybe it was. I am alive because I did have it. I am still recovering and have health to regain, but I'm good. I'm not sure I could've had surgery without support. You were it.

I know you don't really know me, and you probably didn't mean to be so important to me. But you are. I just wanted you to know you were a divine vehicle for me, and I am so grateful to you for being present for that.

Alive and well and healing. Thank you.

• • •

Danny,

It was kind of you to talk with me about surgery. Although I could not afford you, you told me that if surgery had a 95% cure rate (the statistics given me), I should do it. All the energy my body was using to fight cancer might return and be used to live and be well. I leaned on that meeting to accept the cancer treatment. It is no small thing because I did not want surgery.

The surgeon found two cancers, one a super evil aggressive cancer (the surgeon's words), which he removed along with some of my parts. But I am cured, cancer free, healed and healing. 100%. No chemo, no radiation.

Vision, Eyes

Dear Danny,

First, I want to thank you for my miracle. I can't believe that after so many years and so many doctors and so much medication that acupuncture with you was the cure. My eyes feel brand-new again. It is so good to be able to look at a ceiling light without pain and other obstacles.

I thank God for the day I came to you because I can truthfully say, I feel good again. Thank you again and again from the bottom of my heart. You gave me back the most precious thing in life.

P.S. My colitis is about an eight on a scale from 1 to 10, which is a great improvement.

• • •

Dear Dr. Quaranto,

I thank Jill for referring me to you for treatment of my eye nerve jumping. I had been to several doctors who gave me so many pills that I lost count.

After each of your treatments I was great for several days at a time. I can't thank you enough. Turns out I had a bad case of Benign Essential Blepharospasm. If my face starts acting up, I'll be back in your office for more treatment.

Thank you so very much Danny. I tell everyone that acupuncture does help.

Other Ailments

Colitis

Dr. Dan,

Thank you for insisting I try the Gluten Sensitivity Packs. These have seriously changed my life. Coupled with the SCD diet (Paleo), this nutrient-packed daily keeps me normal. Having also colitis for 10 years I never thought I'd get better.

Thank you from the bottom of my heart!

Depression and Anxiety

To whom it may concern:

I am taking this opportunity to express my appreciation for acupuncture services provided by Dr. Danny Quaranto. I was suffering from depression and anxiety, along with the associated symptoms of lack of energy, and loss of appetite and taste. Within two days of an acupuncture treatment for neurotransmitters, I experienced a dramatic improvement that occurred too close to the treatment to be mere coincidence. In addition, a potential thyroid deficiency was uncovered that was missed by traditional blood test. I am sold on alternative medicine, especially as employed by this practitioner. Dr. Quaranto is a valuable health resource for the Vero Beach community.

Dizzy spells and neck tension

Dear Danny,

Since my appointment with you, I have meant to write note of thanks for working me into your tight schedule the day I had the dizzy spells. I had great results from the treatment. Over the past 15 years, I have had regular acupuncture, massage, and homeopathic treatments. You have a calming, healing touch. A good doctor deserves to hear this along with a patient's ailments.

I look forward to seeing you soon after this stressful citrus season. The treatment you gave me for neck tension (the scraping with the spoon) although painful, had miraculous and immediate results.

Thank you again.

Pregnancy

Dear Dr. Quaranto,

Thank you for everything you did to help me. I really think your treatments helped me get pregnant. All is going well!

Severe cough

Dear Danny,

Thank you for the licorice root and your concern. The licorice root helped *a lot*, but the cough was so severe that it did not alleviate it like the other times. I thought I was going to die coughing, but your remedy helped.

I hope we see you soon. Our lives are blessed because we know you. Love

Incontinence

Dear Danny,

You have helped me tremendously. I have not had

any trouble with incontinence since your treatments. It is so embarrassing and I did not relish having to wear Depends the rest of my life.

Then there was the day I could not stop crying because of depression. I walked out of your office laughing.

Now you are helping me with angina, and so far so good. I'd recommend you to anyone, as you know I already do.

Tendonitis

I would like to share an experience I had so others may benefit by having a positive open-minded attitude regarding their health.

About a year and a half ago I was diagnosed with tendinitis in both of my wrists. As anyone with this problem may know, it is very painful and prevents you from doing the simplest of tasks, such as brushing your teeth and changing your child's diaper.

I had physical therapy and wore a brace on one wrist. After several months of treatment and high medical bills, surgery was recommended. I was not comfortable with this and decided to research and explore other methods of treatment.

I met with a prominent local acupuncture expert, Dr. Danny Quaranto. After seven visits, my problem disappeared and has not resurfaced! I also returned for other problems, as well as other family members, all treated with success. He and his staff provided me with the finest care and effective treatment.

I encourage others to be open-minded to alternative ways of treating health problems. For enjoyable healthcare with positive results, educate yourself and seek other opinions, even if they are considered "alternative." Alternative" may be the way to go.

Tinnitus

Dear Dr. Quaranto,

I have been your patient for a number of years. During that time you have helped me a great deal to achieve better health.

You helped heal my tinnitus, the ringing in my ears, which drove me crazy. In addition, you help me with phlegm and breathing issues. You also counseled me on proper nutrition. And you treated me for a variety of pains and medical issues.

I greatly appreciate and respect your medical care. Sincerely.

Multitude of issues

Dear Dr. Quaranto,

The other day I was thinking how much the acupuncture and herbs have helped me. I want you to know how grateful I am for this.

As you will recall, I came initially for only asthma, but I'm happy to say there is a long list of other ailments that you have helped me with.

Asthma: Allergy shots, asthma insulators, and pills gave me only partial relief. Now I can walk at a good pace for an hour without any wheezing or puffing. Also, during a severe attack when I could not get my breath, you applied needles in just the right locations and the spasm quieted immediately, and I could breathe once more.

Arthritis: My hips and knees are painful. And because I am drug sensitive, I can take only Tylenol. Now I can be on my knees without pain and I don't even take Tylenol.

Energy: The acupuncture has raised my energy level to the point I just keep going all day without a nap, bright-eyed and bushy-tailed as the saying goes.

Alertness, concentration, and memory: Before the treatments I lacked the concentration and memory to play a good game of bridge. I even found it difficult to read more than a very simple novel. Now I give my bridge partner is a challenge and enjoy reading whatever I choose.

Feet: I have Morton's Neuroma, which is painful on both feet. For years doctors have advised surgery. Now I am on my feet for hours without pain and wear nice looking shoes without discomfort.

Scalp: Three years ago a beautician burnt my head with permanent lotion causing my scalp to have rashes, pustules, and scabs. Two dermatologists prescribed five lotions and shampoos which did not help. One acupuncture treatment was all it took to heal my scalp.

Digestion: For about eight years I have been able to eat only fish and no other meat. This in spite of food allergy shots and numerous stomach medicines. I now eat all meats because of herbs and acupuncture.

Sinus: You are working on this still, but it has greatly improved.

Allergies: For years I've had severe allergies with exotic reactions despite allergy shots. I'm about 90% improved.

Fever: I can hardly believe I even had fever. Your treatment has brought me back to normal.

Heart racing and pounding: I don't know why this

happened, and doctors did not know why or how to stop it. My racing, pounding heart would keep me awake, but it rarely happens now since the acupuncture treatments.

Sleep: For 14 years I didn't have a single night's good sleep. Some nights I would not sleep at all. That's no fun! I took sleeping pills but stopped because of doctor's advice. Now, after your treatments, 90% of the time I sleep well. I can't describe how marvelous this is.

Skin: My shins were dry, itchy, and bleeding from scratching. Also, my knees were scaly and white. Thanks to acupuncture the skin is now normal. Also, my lips were so chapped that they would bleed. I seldom experienced this now.

Please feel free to show this letter to new patients. I would be glad to talk with them about it if they would like. I know this will embarrass you because you are a humble man. But I find you a kind, caring, and compassionate physician.

Sincerely and gratefully yours.

Wondrous Healing

Once again, I thank you for my daughter's improved health. I was pleased with her progress one year ago when I was in Florida. But now I am more than impressed! It's like a miracle! You have accomplished what dozens of other's could not.

Thank you for your persistence and for taking her seriously. May you be as successful with all your patients.

• • •

Table of Contents

Thank you Danny so very much. The many healings occurring within me are wondrous. I'm profoundly grateful for the changes your work facilitated within me. I appreciate your dedication, training, and willingness to share. Be well.

My problem improved dramatically

My treatment at The Acupuncture Center of Vero Beach was pleasant and beneficial. My problem improved dramatically, although it was not completely eliminated— at least not yet. I expect to be cured when I return for treatment after the demands on my time have ended.

Thank you for your patience, and congratulations on the quality of treatment, as well as the concern for your patients.

Making Life Worthwhile

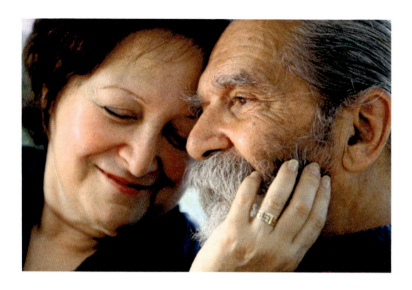

Dr. Danny received his medical degree (MD) in June 2015. Some of these letters reflect this milestone.

Now I Smile

I want to thank you for the smiles I smiled all day just thinking about it. For the way the world looks better to me because you brightened it. And for the warmth I feel because I know someone cares.

Your thoughtfulness touched my life in more ways than you know.

Kindness

Danny,

Thank you so much for all you've done, by not only your services and talents but also your kindness through a difficult time.

Now I have a Vision

Dear Dr. Quaranto,

Thank you so much for allowing me to spend two days at your office. You and your staff were so generous in sharing your knowledge, experience, and time.

I left your office yesterday feeling inspired and excited about practicing alternative medicine. The way you practice—your inclusion of so many healing modalities; your manner and demeanor with your patients, staff and me; your business practices—gave me a foundation for a vision of what my own practice can be.

Back to Health and Balance

Dear Dr. Danny,

You have been my health inspiration and my guide to better health and happiness for many years. I respect and honor your health knowledge, your passion to help others, and your desire to do your best. Thank you so much for helping me return to a healthy and balanced life.

Congratulations on your MD degree. Thank you and bless you always.

Don't Ever Leave Vero

Dear Dr. Danny,

Congratulations to an awesome doc! Wow, is there anything you can't do? We loved seeing your graduation festivities on Facebook. We are so proud of you and happy you reached another of your many goals. I guess it is what keeps you so "young."

You have done absolute wonders for my family and

me. So glad we are now lifelong friends. Every time one of us has a crisis, your expertise, and careful guidance has pulled us through.

Don't ever leave Vero or you will have tons of patients (including me) following you around the world.

Love and hugs.

You Have Changed My Life

Dr. Danny,

Congratulations! You are truly an inspiration of a man following his dream and accomplishing what he sets out to do. I am blessed to have found you; how you have changed my life! You are dearly loved for desiring to help so many in the quest for better.

Congrats. I'm so happy for you. Love you.

The Most Amazing Doctor

Dr. Danny,

Congratulations! You are amazing, how you love to heal and know what's best. You are our guru,☺ the most marvelous doctor in the whole world.

We love you Dr. Danny.

You Are an Inspiration

Dear Dr. Danny,

You are an incredible inspiration and your mastery of Eastern and Western medicine is remarkable. Thank you for all you have done for me and my family and my friends. I feel blessed to have you in my life. I wish you all the best always.

You Did It!

Dr. Danny,

Well you did it! I'm so happy for you. It was a long road and you were determined.

My time here has been and still is helping me getting my body back on track.

Congratulations again; so glad that I have been here to see you finish your studies and reach this landmark in your life.

All the best.

A Man Following His Dreams

Dr. Danny,

Congrats. You are truly an inspiration, a man following his dreams and accomplishing what he sets out to achieve. I am blessed to have found you. How you have changed my life and that of my family. You're dearly loved by our family and treasured desiring to help so many in the quest for long and better health. Congrats-praise God! Love.

A Legend in Our Family's Life

Dr. Danny,

You are an inspiration and a blessing to our lives. The changes we experienced with our health—mind, body, and spirit—are profound.

Thank you for always being there to help, and your willingness to tackle the toughest tasks. You are legend in our family's life. We hope your saga continues for many years to come!

We love you.

Living and enjoying life

Dear Danny,

Hi! Just a quick note to say hello and thanks for helping my father out with his back. I just got off the phone with him and he was *elated* with the results of your treatment!

You have helped everyone I sent to you. I'm glad I found you back in November. I know you can help me with breathing and relaxation techniques. I haven't had any neck problems since I came to you either!

A Man For All Five Seasons*

A Well Rounded and Balanced Personality

It's not so much what a person says or teaches, nor his perfection, that makes him stand tall. Rather, it's the symmetry of his character, its balanced unification.

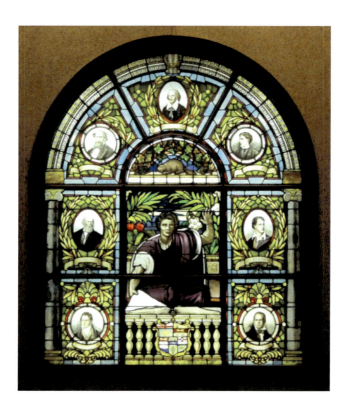

---

* The Fifth Season is approximately a two week transition period between the four traditional seasons.

Family Man

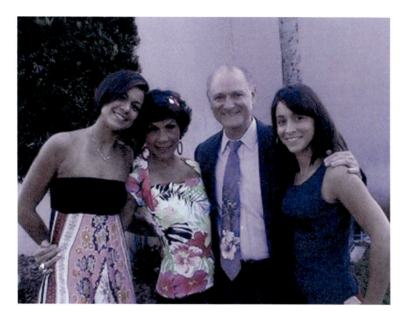

Dr. Danny, wife Josefina, daughters
Danielle and Adriana

At play

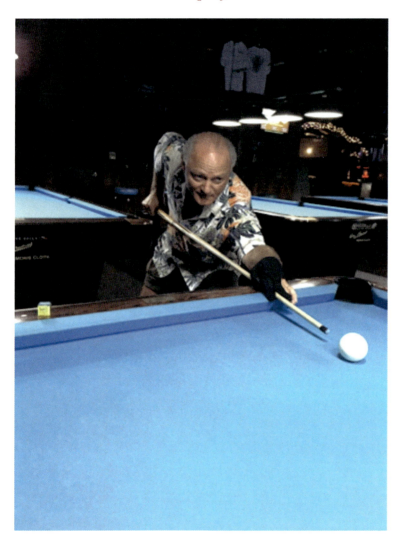

Dr. Danny is a serious pool player.

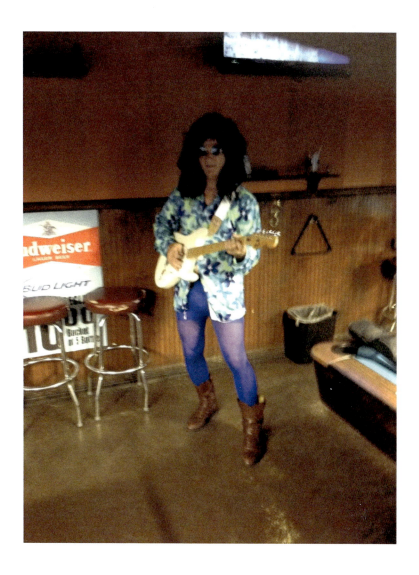

Yes! It is Dr. Danny as his alter ego known as *Essence*. It's healthy not to take yourself too seriously, don't you think?

Ever learning and healing

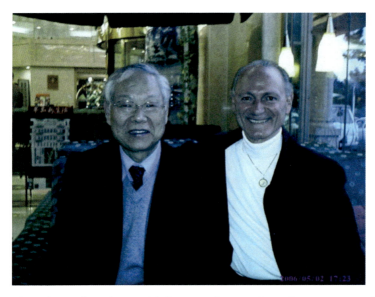

Dr. Zhu in Qingdao, China, where Dr. Danny worked with him in the Neurology Ward of the Affiliated Hospital of the Qingdao Medical School. They treated stroke patients solely with scalp acupuncture.

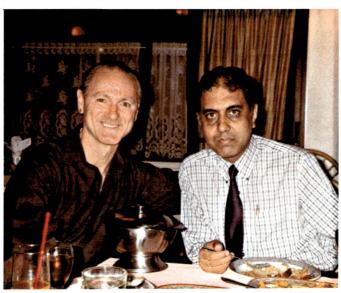

Dr. Danny & Master Homeopath & Friend Dr. Subrata Kumar Banerjea

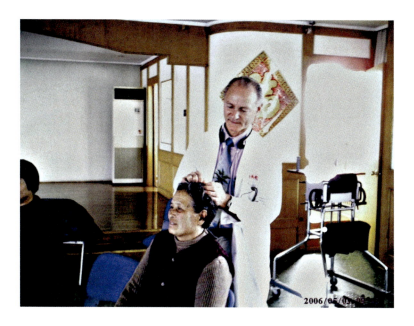

Performing scalp acupuncture on a patient in Qingdao

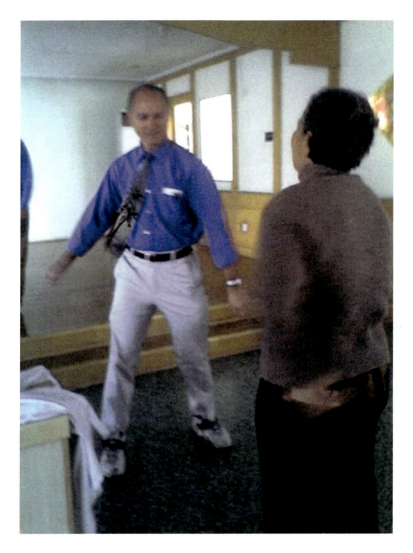

Treating stroke patients at the neurology ward of the Affiliated Hospital of the Qingdao Medical School

Martial arts

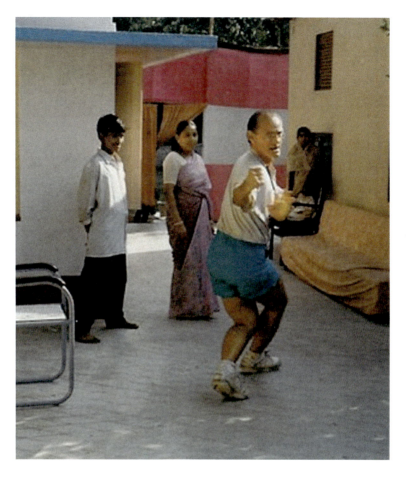

Demonstrating Kung Fu in the Calcutta slums

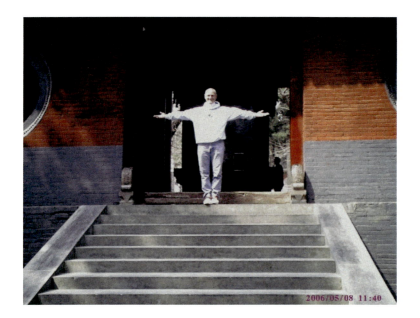

Dr. Danny at a Shaolin Temple in China, a center for martial arts. And there is another story of traveling through China alone without a translator. Adventure anyone?

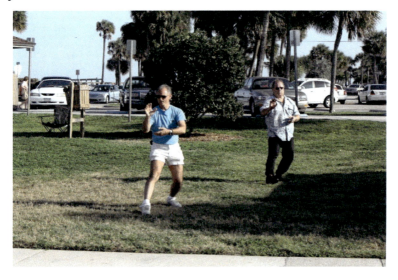

Teaching Tai Chi at Jaycee Park

Teacher

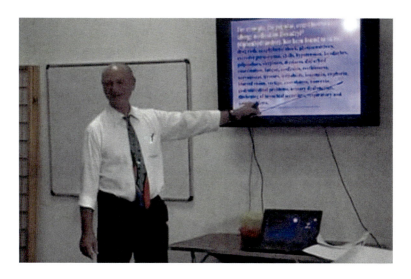

Dr. Danny teaches free classes on common ailments

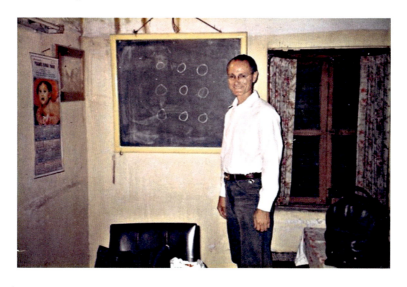

Teaching in Calcutta

Traveler

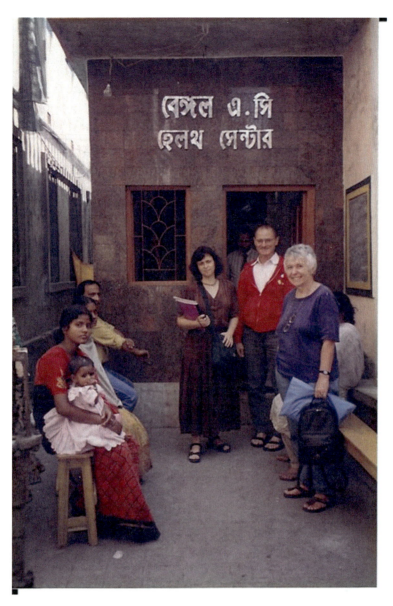

In the Calcutta slums

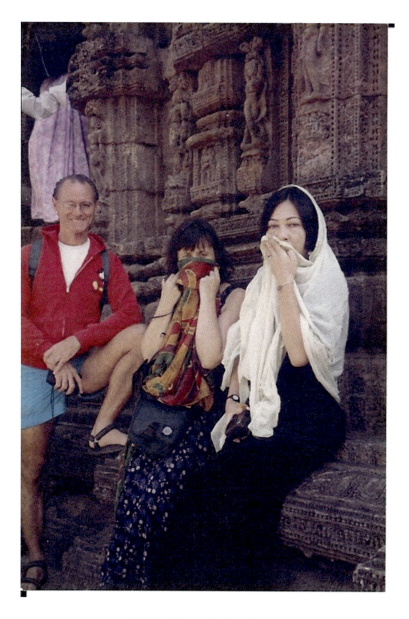

With friends in Calcutta

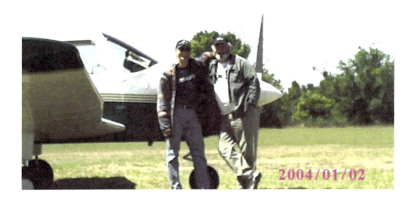

Dr. Danny the pilot and Chris flying into Chalet Suzanne for breakfast

Speaking to groups

Thank you again for taking the time to talk to our group, Surviving Spouses. Many members, including myself, share a deep interest in alternative healing techniques. The mind-body connection is fascinating and we all appreciate the talk you gave. Warmest regards.

Conclusion of the matter

As a tree is known by its fruit, so has alternative medicine blossomed the lives of my patients, nurturing them from barren branches to ripened fruit, living lives once again rewarding and fulfilling.

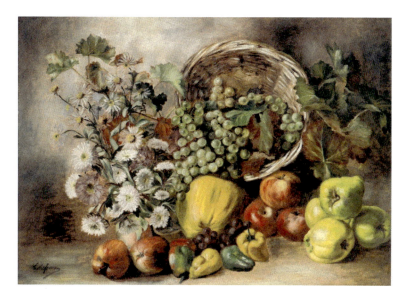

Come and dine!

A Patient Sums it Up

Dear Dr. Quaranto,

You explained how you work the very first time I met you. One thought stood out and remains indelible: When you studied in China, you learned that a healer considers he has failed if his patients become sick. Wow! I never had a doctor tell me that!

You explained that your job is to prevent the body from losing its harmony so symptoms finally appear—the tip of the iceberg. In China, patients go regularly for a "tune-up," (my way of putting it) so a budding disharmony is corrected before it becomes a disease.

You suggested quarterly checkups after first returning my body to a state of harmony. It made sense and I gladly schedule my tune-ups, not only for prevention or correcting what may have cropped up since my last visit, but also to say hi and share and laugh with you.

As I've come to know you, it's delightful to see the balanced life you lead, things others may not know about you. You play the guitar, are an avid chess player, play 3-cushion billiards, and play pool at a team level—and I'm sure there's more. This is in addition to publicly teaching, conducting Tai Chi, and continually educating yourself because it is your delight to know more.

There are those in every community who are assets, most of whom remain unknown except for those who benefit directly. You are a treasure to our small county on the Treasure Coast.

Well done Doctor Danny. You are a Man for All Seasons.

Taking Control of your Health

This is written by Richard Rosen, one of my patients. It makes the point of how crucial it is to become responsible for your own health and not delegate decision making to another.

Live healthy to maximize spirituality

Take control of your health. Pollutions of the physical body retard the efforts of the Indwelling Spirit to raise the level of mind beyond the merely natural. A healthy lifestyle promotes a sound body that supports spiritual achievement.

> The (Indwelling Spirit) remains with you in all disaster and through every sickness which does not wholly destroy the mentality. But how unkind knowingly to defile or otherwise deliberately to pollute the physical body, which must serve as the earthly tabernacle of this marvelous gift from God.
>
> All physical poisons greatly retard the efforts of the Adjuster to exalt the material mind while the mental poisons of fear, anger, envy, jealousy, suspicion, and intolerance likewise tremendously interfere with the spiritual progress of the evolving soul. (Urantia Book, 110:1.5, p.1204¶3)

I am a believer that most difficulties are of our own making. There are things outside of our control, such as heredity and natural disaster, but even these can be made the best of. We create the environment in which we live and our health improves or deteriorates accordingly.

We have become a chemical society. What I mean is

that the chemical industry has become ubiquitous in the products we eat, put on our skin and breathe. Chronic end-of-life diseases that plague most elderly people in developed countries are in large part caused by decades of ingesting chemicals and exposure to a toxic environment. Mix in a little more MSG? How about a wee bit of yellow dye? Ugh!

I asked my alternative medical practitioner about a skin lotion, showing him the ingredients. There were more than a dozen chemical formulations, most of which could not be pronounced. He took one look and said, "As a rule of thumb, if you cannot pronounce it, don't eat it or put it on your skin." And neither would I breathe it, which means from such sources as cleaning supplies, secondhand smoke or air polluted cities that you can avoid visiting— and certainly think twice about living there.

We each need to take control of our health by making our own medical decisions with the input from practitioners who share our viewpoint, all the while researching on our own those things needful to maintain a sound and healthy body—which is the foundation of intelligent thinking, emotional well-being, and ultimately, spiritual growth. Here is an example:

I had been taking hormones to balance out things. I took blood tests for my next appointment and it turned out my doctor did not include these particular hormones for testing. I had relied upon him to include them. In his busyness he did not and so I had to take another blood test.

It made me realize that it was my responsibility to check everything, not only to ensure what should be present is there, but also to make suggestions for other things that may be appropriate. Moreover, I recognized that as I gain more knowledge that I need not consult with him on all things, having gained the wisdom to know when I could do things on my own. A doctor can be viewed as a trusted professional with whom you share ideas and value his expertise and counsel. But he better share your point of view on health.

The human race is susceptible to many illnesses and diseases. Things can be done to minimize contracting them, such as washing your hands and avoiding the presence of sick people or taking precautions when in their presence. Take control.

These are the main things that determine health in my view:

- Nutrition, including the highest quality vitamin and mineral supplements
- Exercise
- Minimized exposure to environmental toxins
- Correct posture
- Reduction of stress
- Knowledge of alternative medical solutions coupled with awareness of the limitations and dangers of conventional medicine.

Educate yourself to maintain your health

With the poor ethics practiced by business today, companies will often manufacture health products and deliver health services they either know are unhealthy or they choose to remain willfully ignorant of in the pursuit of profit. Think of the tobacco industry; then apply the same mindset to what I'd dare say is every industry.

The Complementary and Alternative Medicine (CAM) movement that promotes non-conventional wellness solutions has risen in protest. The same is happening in other industries, but generally, it is smaller businesses that choose ethical solutions. Once a company has lost the ethical vision and drive of its original founders, the widespread mentality of profit above all takes hold. Vitiated products and service invariably follow.

It's wise—no, it's crucial—to research alternative views about maintaining wellness and dealing with specific heath issues. With the Internet that information is now readily accessible. I strongly recommend www.mercola.com as a source of health-related information. I research questions I have there and educate myself with their daily email newsletter.

Alternative medicine solutions

I began my education in alternative medicine in the early 90s by reading books of Dr. Andrew Weil. From him I learned that foundational to healthy living is understanding that the body is designed to heal itself; you just need to remove the poisons that prevent it, whether from what you eat or the environment or your mind and emotions.

There is a large array of alternative health solutions, enough to become bewildered; which do I choose? Each lays out a path to the summit of health. Each reaches the peak from a different side of the mountain on its uniquely configured path. Each of us must decide which solutions align best with who we are. They all ascend the same height, of not merely good, but optimal health.

My research of a subject includes the experiences of others. That provides an authenticity of actual experience that complements the scientific and marketing claims of a health solution or product.

Alternative care as a financial investment

Many are deterred from using alternative health practitioners and products because insurance covers few of them. You pay it all.

From my experience, it's first necessary to understand and believe your health and well-being will substantially improve to justify the cost. It begins as a faith effort until you come to "know" the truth of the matter. At the beginning of this journey you must swim upstream against the current, the mindset of the vast majority of institutions and the general population. The primary cause of this adverse current is the determined obstructionism to alternative medical care from the conventional medical complex (defined below).

My experience is that it costs less over time to pay out of pocket compared with insurance paid conventional disease management (not prevention and optimal health mind you). How is this so? Foremost, you avoid a diseased body and becoming a ward of the medical system. What is feeling well worth to you?

Secondly, because you remain healthy you will have avoided illness and the often considerable expense associated with it. For example, my brother spent one night in the hospital and left with an $1100 bill—and that's with Medicare and supplemental health insurance. That would have paid for a lot of alternative medical care. And what about lost wages and productivity from ill health you avoid?

But when it's all said and done, improved health and quality of life justify the expense, learning, and effort to countervail the culture of conventional medicine.

• • •

For those interested in the application of spiritual principles to daily living, Richard Rosen's *Living Spiritually* series includes:

Life After Death:
A step by step account of what happens next

Dear Abba:
God answers heartfelt problems of everyday living

Living Spiritually in a Practical World:
How to attune yourself to divine guidance

About the Author

All too often it's the doctor who gets all the information about the patient, and the patient gets little information about the doctor and his or her practice. As with many things in medicine, it needs changing, which this introduction does.

My name is Danny Quaranto and I was born in West Newton, MA on February 18, 1949. I hold a Medical Degree from the University of Science, Arts and Technology—Montserrat, Caribbean. I graduated from the New England School of Acupuncture (N.E.S.A.) on June 6, 1986. I am certified by the National Commission for the Certification of Acupuncture and Oriental Medicine (N.C.C.A.O.M.) in both Acupuncture and Chinese Herbal Medicine.

The joys of my life are my wife, Josefina, who teaches me through example that my greatness is limited only by my imagination, and two young women named, Danielle and Adriana, whom I am honored to call my daughters. I have been practicing Kung Fu and Tai Chi since 1973 and hold free classes open to the public every Sunday at 5:00PM at Jaycee Park, Vero Beach. I also enjoy meditating, playing tennis, basketball, pool, and chess, and I am an instrument-rated pilot of single engine airplanes.

I was originally inspired to become a Doctor of Oriental Medicine through my love and immersion in all aspects of the Chinese martial arts. An important part of Kung Fu teaches that if you hurt yourself or someone else, you should be able to take care of that injury. In my quest to learn more and to become proficient in this healing aspect of the martial arts, I jumped into acupuncture school with both feet and began an amazing dynamic journey that will continue for the rest of my life.

Part of this journey included an internship at the Affiliated Hospital of Qingdao University Medical School, Qingdao, China, where I worked in the neurology department specializing in the treatment of post-stroke patients.

Through my endless continuing studies I was introduced to Classical Homeopathy. This immense study led me to Calcutta, India to receive advanced clinical training at the Bengal Allen Medical Institute. Interestingly, Oriental Medicine and Classical Homeopathy are based on the same energetic principles.

I've chosen to devote my life to the healing arts because I have a gift and a passion to share with the world, an awareness that we need to trust the life force that is the only thing that ever heals us. My highest and only calling is to help sick people become well and to help them become ready and willing to help themselves. I am eternally grateful that I devoted myself to the healing arts because I continually experience the magnificent miracle of life on a tangible daily basis. I get excited watching people get rid of the limitations that keep them from being connected to vital force and balance in their lives. Mental clarity and emotional stability without physical limitations are the ideal. In a word, a patient's "freedom" is my goal.

I believe with all of my heart in the principles of Oriental Medicine, which state that the power that made the body can also heal the body. All dis-ease is the result of a blockage in the flow of that life force that allows our bodily processes to function as they should. These blockages are both caused by and can cause mental, emotional or physical symptoms.

I also deeply believe in how I practice Alternative Medicine, and I constantly strive to improve my God-given talent. I believe I give an excellent service for a fair price. I want to help people. I want you to refer and continue to refer patients to me because the more people that experience holistic care, the healthier the entire world will be. This creates a ripple effect where one person affects one family, which in turn affects one community, one state, one continent, one world, and eventually one universe.

The reason that I came to beautiful Vero Beach and established the Acupuncture Center of Vero Beach in 1989 is that it was a perfect place to raise my children. Additionally, the higher level of consciousness in Vero Beach has always seemed fertile ground to plant the seeds of awareness that Alternative Medicine must be a first choice option for health care. Many people over the years have asked me, "When I'm having a problem, how do I know if I need to see you or my conventional doctor?" My answer is, "If you don't have to call 911, you can call me." Always explore the least invasive form of medicine first. If we decide that your condition warrants more heroic measures, you will be referred to an appropriate healthcare provider."

The mission of the Center is to help as many people as possible in their quest for optimal health and to educate those people so they in turn can educate others about the benefits of Alternative Medicine. We wish to provide Alternative Medicine to our community as a first choice option to help you regain your health. My desire is that people receive and learn care for the entire person (body, mind, emotions, and spirit) with this wonderful comprehensive form of medicine that is safe and effective for everyone, including pregnant women, infants, and elderly people, without the use of drugs or surgery.

What makes this practice unique is the synthesis of many technologies to maximize the patient's ultimate potential. These include the nine major branches of Oriental Medicine as well as other therapies.

- Acupuncture and Chinese Herbs
- Classical Homeopathy in the tradition of Hahnemann
- Neuro-Emotional Technique (NET™)
- Neuro-Emotional Anti-sabotage Technique (N.E.A.T)
- Natural Allergy Elimination Technique
- Enzyme Replacement Therapy (E.R.T.)
- Jaffe-Mellor Technique (JMT)
- Neuro-Modulation Technique (NMT™)
- Acupoint Injection Therapy
- Prolotherapy
- Apitherapy
- Bio-Cranial Therapy
- Nutritional and Lifestyle Counseling
- Functional Neurology

Because acupuncture itself is a growing and dynamic part of Oriental Medicine, many modern, gentle, and effective techniques have developed. Therefore, if you choose not to experience traditional acupuncture needling during treatment, I can use other safe and effective methods to help you without using the hair-thin, painless needles.

Here is what I promise you: I will do everything in my power to lead you to optimum health and freedom on every level. I realize that this is a new experience for many people so I welcome your questions. I look forward to a lifelong relationship with you and I congratulate you for choosing this office for your health care needs.

Acknowledgements

Words fail to express the heartfelt gratitude I feel toward so many for having taken the time to teach and encourage me over the years.

First, I want to give special thanks to my wife, Josefina, for loving and trusting me enough to give me free reign to build a life of purpose and caring, especially the decision to teach martial arts for a living—and then to become an acupuncturist in the early 1980s, a time when acupuncture was not as popular as it is now. All this with the added challenge of raising two daughters who at the time were 4 and 5 years old. You are a Saint.

I would also like to express my gratitude to Richard Rosen who conceived the idea for this book and mobilized the Qi to bring it to fruition. You are truly a talented and creative man and an author in your own right, having written three books.

Of course, without patient testimonials, we would not have a book. I am humbled when I read patients' comments and am awed by the power of this medicine that has allowed me to witness so many miracles. Thank you so much for sharing your unsolicited stories. It is an inspiration to me and to others.

This life journey began at the Wah Lum Kung Fu Academy in Boston in 1973 under the tutelage of Master Chan Pui, who accepted me as a 7th generation disciple into the Wah Lum system. He taught me that if, as a martial arts practitioner, you are injured, or you injure someone else, then you should be able to take care of that injury. I was always intrigued with that aspect of Chinese martial arts and when I had the opportunity to go to acupuncture school, I closed my Kung Fu school and dove into acupuncture school to begin the endless journey. I thank Master Chan for the Dit Da Jow (Hit Fall Wine) formula that I continuously use in my medical practice.

I have had many incredible teachers who have helped me acquire skills and techniques which have helped thousands of suffering patients. One such teacher was Taoist monk, Ken Cohen, who taught me that "when your heart is pure, the gods ride on the needle, and every point is an acupuncture point." This taught me that intention is as important as technique.

I thank Iva Lim Peck from the bottom of my heart for introducing me to muscle testing and allergy elimination, both of which revolutionized my practice and provided a vehicle for me to explain to patients why they were feeling the way that they feel. If muscle testing technology had been available to Sun Si Miao and Samuel Hahnemann it would have changed the whole complexion of Chinese Medicine and Homeopathy.

I thank Datis Kharrazian, DC for blowing my mind. I would walk out of a Datis seminar with my head spinning with the possibilities that he opened up for me to help more sick people to get well.

I thank Scott Walker, DC for teaching me Neuro-Emotional Technique (NET), a revolutionary technique that allows me to access and eliminate the blockages that keep us all from doing, being, and having whatever it is that we want to do, be, and have, and also to extinguish the physiology of emotions that perpetuate our physical ailments.

I thank the numerous talented instructors of the Naturopathic Association of Therapeutic Injections, for placing into my tool box an incredible treatment

(Prolotherapy, aka Regenerative Injection Therapy), which helps to rebuild and restore the integrity of connective tissue.

I would like to thank Thea Elijah, DOM for the enlightened perspective on the spirit and properties of Chinese herbal medicine that only she is able to convey.

I would like to thank Edwin Floyd, DC for inspiring me to go further in my homeopathic studies.

I would like to thank my friend and mentor Dr. Subrata Kumar Banerjea for fine tuning my homeopathic education in the slums of Calcutta, India, an experience I could receive nowhere else in the world. It demonstrated the infinite power of homeopathic medicine. All Praise to Samuel Hahnemann, MD.

Thank you so much to Mingqing Zhu, DOM for showing me the power of scalp acupuncture to help those suffering from the after effects of strokes. I saw people in China who, after having had a stroke and not being able to walk or speak, were able to get out of a wheelchair and read a newspaper out loud after two days of treatment using Dr. Zhu's system of scalp acupuncture.

Thank you to my dear friend, Kate Hoffmann, DOM, AP for generously agreeing to write the Forward in this edition.

Thank you to Lee Funk, MD, DOM, DC who lovingly badgered me into applying to medical school.

Thank you to all of the wonderful doctors with whom I did my clinical training for medical school. They are Orion Tulp, MD Kenneth Director, MD, John Sarbak, MD, Felix Bigay, MD, George Fyffe, MD, Deni Malave, MD, Cristina Dupree, DO, and especially Terry Swezey MD who has cared for me and my family since 1989. He is a true teacher and I thank him for his generosity in sharing his knowledge.

Thank you to my mentor at medical school, Bruce Robinson, MD who taught me the power of loving your patients and treating them with patience and compassion.

On the shoulders of these great people I gratefully and humbly stand.

Public Teaching and Health Videos

These free one-hour workshops introduce remedies of common problems.
- Natural Solutions and Prevention of Arthritis
- How to Eliminate Allergies Naturally
- Lowering Cholesterol: Get the Facts
- Autoimmune Disorders: Why are You Killing Yourself?
- Natural Solutions to Anxiety and Depression
- Natural Solutions to Gastrointestinal Problems
- Natural Solutions to Cardiovascular Problems
- Headaches & Migraines (coming soon!)
- Diabetes
- Hormones
- Acupressure
- The Story Your Blood Tells About You

You can view videos of these teachings at www.amfcc.info/classes.html.

Made in the USA
Columbia, SC
23 June 2021